weight loss
the forgotten secret

42 powerful ways to get slim and
stay slim with the new self-hypnosis

cus D'Silva

Weight loss the forgotton secret

Published by New London Publishing Ltd

Copyright © Marcus D`Silva 2007

British library cataloguing in publication data a catalogue record for this book is available from the British library

Cover design by Mark Richardson

I.S.B.N No 0-9554446-0-8

Printed in Great Britain by
Antony Rowe Ltd, Chippenham, Wiltshire

*I dedicate this book
to my wonderful wife
Deborah*

Contents

Introduction
Diets don't work!

Diets don't work! Introduction

How many times have you found yourself being seduced by the latest fresh-out-of-the oven diet plan?

The fact that you are reading this book tells me you have probably in the past fallen prey to some of the many so-called magic pills or diets of the weight-loss industry.

It has been stated (quite accurately) that 95% of weight-loss diets fail, so what is the key to reducing your weight and keeping it off? You are soon to find out.

In my own personal experience with controlling my own weight I have probably tried 80% of all the so-called diets on the market, including living on rice cakes for six weeks!

Now don't get me wrong. Most of these diets do create weight loss, and a few are worth studying, but, as far as keeping it off and feeling good about yourself inside, something is clearly missing.

If diets worked, you would only have to do it once, right?

You may notice that the harder you try to keep to a diet the more difficult it becomes. This is because will power is not the right approach to lasting weight loss.

Here is a quick exercise that demonstrates just what I mean.

Close your eyes and try not to think about the colour red. For most of you it is almost impossible because you have to access a visual representation of the colour red to understand what I am talking about. It is like the more you tell yourself "I will try not to eat chocolate" the more you reinforce the behaviour.
Remember trying is lying.

Too many people focus on what they don't want instead of what they do want. Through using your mind as the main tool for reaching your ideal weight, you can literally think yourself slim.

There are people who strongly believe that they can eat what they want and stay slim, and they can, because the strength of their beliefs creates behaviours to match. You may think of it as a self- fulfilling prophecy. In other words if you change your beliefs, behaviour change will follow.

Go out and speak to people who say they can eat what they want and stay slim. What beliefs do they hold about themselves? Beg steal or borrow those beliefs. It will help get you started on the road to becoming your ideal weight.

The fight for your mind!

Marketing experts are clever. They know just how to position themselves in your mind through advertising and marketing.

We are all constantly being influenced by others in many areas of our lives, including by our friends and family. Persuasion and influence are facts of life, but you can learn to influence yourself. You don't have to be a robot that becomes re-active to every new weight loss diet or product that is put on the market to whet your appetite. You can learn to win the fight of your own mind through self hypnosis and following some simple weight-loss rules.

In this book you will learn how to see yourself at your ideal weight; learn to accept yourself unconditionally; learn how to identify emotional eating; learn the truth about diet and exercise, and programme yourself for success.

Your ideal body is sleeping in your own mind right now! It's time to wake it up.

How to use his book

To get the most out of this book, read it through from cover to cover. Then go back to the beginning and start to work through the different sections.

It is important that you spend time working only with the trance inductions for the first 2 weeks. This will help release tension and stress from your body and help you focus your mind.

After you feel comfortable with the basic trance inductions, move on to the awareness and acceptance sections, developing these skills over a further 2 week period, slowly integrating them into your daily trance practice. The next step is to move on to the self- image section. This is the core work of changing your mental blueprint - the way you see yourself.

By the time you have developed these skills over a total period of 4-6 weeks, you will feel calmer, more relaxed, more in tune with your inner nature and you will find those extra pounds beginning to melt away.

You are now ready to start experimenting with the other approaches in this book.

You will find powerful techniques for controlling emotional eating, increasing motivation, resolving inner conflicts and eliminating chocolate addictions.

You will learn how to re-frame negative thinking, break unwanted behaviour patterns, and use your mind to programme new habits and behaviours, helping you to achieve lasting weight loss.

Have fun!

"You go into self-hypnosis to achieve certain things or acquire certain knowledge "

- Erickson and Rossi 1977

1. What is Self Hypnosis?

Believe it or not, it is a natural gift that lies within us; we were all born to use the power of our minds.

Through the centuries many great men and women have learned how to tap into their inner potential to achieve outstanding results in their lives. Self hypnosis is the bridge to our subconscious minds. It has been suggested that we only use about 10% of our brain, not something we should be bragging about.

Hypnosis taps into the other 90% - exactly how much who knows, Perhaps hundreds of years ago these natural human powers were more evident, but over the years as our world has become more and more stressful, we have somehow lost touch with this ability. The actual terms for hypnosis come under many guises - relaxation, visualisation, inner focus, meditation, mental imagery and altered states. Anyone who has experienced any of the above has been into hypnosis.

Is hypnosis safe? The truth

Occasionally people ask me if hypnosis is safe?

This is not surprising with the many distorted perceptions about hypnosis that have developed over the last century.

The truth is hypnosis (or trance) is a natural phenomenon that we have all experienced many times in our lives.

For those of you who drive, you may have had the experience of driving to a familiar destination and wondered how you got there because you had almost no memory of the journey.

This is because you were on autopilot.

You probably have driven this route so many times you don't need to consciously figure it out.

This is a form of unconscious learning and is an example of a common natural every day trance.

Other examples of this are gazing at a naked flame. After a short time you begin to trance out, so to speak.

You may recall yourself day dreaming, perhaps staring out of a window and feeling like you were miles away (in your imagination)

This too is a natural common every day trance.

Films like the 1931 Svengali starring John Barrymore have not helped.

In the film Barrymore hypnotised young women to carry out evil crimes. Films and books like this almost certainly helped to create a mysterious side to hypnosis. Then came stage hypnosis to make matters even more confusing.

It is worth keeping in mind that stage hypnotists are showmen. They create an illusion, leading people to think they hold some power. Of course this is just a clever form of entertainment.

The truth is hypnosis is part of everyday life.

Marketer's, sales people, politicians, our mothers, fathers, spouses and children all influence us to an extent.

Self-hypnosis as we are using it here is an altered state of awareness. A pleasant comfortable state in which you are open to new positive ideas and suggestions, and are at all times in complete control. You create your own hypnosis.

Your subconscious mind

Before you start practising self-hypnosis, it is useful to have a basic understanding about the subconscious mind.

As young children we spent much of our time in a fantasy world, daydreaming, drifting off into imaginary lands. We had no concept of time; we were creative and fearless, our bodies relaxed and healthy.

As children we spent much of our time in a natural trance state, using more of our subconscious mind, because the subconscious is the part of our mind that generates our feelings and creativity. It has no concept of time, and is non-logical.

As we grow older, we develop more and more of our conscious mind. We start to learn how to tell the time, read, write, think more logically, more rationally. We begin to use more of our conscious minds?

By the time we become adults, many of us become more time-conscious, less creative, more anxious and stressed, and less aware of our inner selves. In a sense as we grow older we also become more and more out of touch with who we really are.

Self-hypnosis is a wonderful tool for getting in touch with our inner selves again, to create changes in our life, by enhancing our creativity, changing unwanted habits and behaviours, eliminating stress and anxiety, and improving our health. Self-hypnosis can help us to experience success and happiness in many areas of our life. Trance is, in a nutshell, going inside and communicating with our subconscious.

How does it feel?

Let's get one thing straight - you are not asleep. 90% of people are completely aware of everything that goes on. Self-hypnosis is a relaxed, meditative, peaceful, comfortable state of mind in which you guide the whole process.

 By going into hypnosis we find all our present beliefs temporarily suspended, allowing us to programme more useful ones so we can move toward our chosen goals in life, in fact we really are de-hypnotising ourselves from negative beliefs and behaviours, letting go of negative programming that no longer serves us.

Self hypnosis and weight control.

Using self hypnosis in weight control can be a powerful way to create new beliefs and to tap into our own inner resources.

I personally in my own clinical practice have seen clients create some amazing changes in their lives through self- hypnosis.

So how can we use our minds to become slimmer, happier and more confident about ourselves?

The secret lies in changing our self-image, the way in which we see ourselves, our own mental blueprint.

People with weight problems almost always drift through life, seeing themselves as over-weight and unattractive.

The core strength of ourselves lies in a positive self-image, which has a big influence on our self- esteem

Self-esteem is a basic need - "it really is alright to love yourself." There are two main components to our self esteem – self-efficacy and self-respect.

Self-efficacy is having confidence in your ability to think, learn, understand, and make decisions in your life.

Self-respect is having assurance of your own self-worth, asserting your wants and needs. Soon you will learn some powerful ways of changing your self-image and improving your self-esteem.

Weight loss and stress.

Things are tough at the office, your credit cards are building up, and you have problems with the car. You get the idea!
While the immediate response to distress is to eat less, it has been found that for many people the opposite is true.

Heavy work loads and long hours can lead to quick fast-food habits, comfort eating and no time for exercise. Guess what? You start to get fatter, you feel terrible and it becomes a vicious circle.

One of the secrets of achieving your ideal weight is learning how to control your stress levels. We will look at how to deal with unwanted stress in a few moments.

How long and where and when?

Self-hypnosis is much like going to the gym or your local health club. It needs to be done on a regular basis to produce good results. Regular exercise will give you a fit, healthy body in a relatively short period of time, if it is done consistently.

This is true for self- hypnosis. Daily trances are recommended for optimum results. You will find after practising self-hypnosis for three to four weeks you will look forward to taking time for yourself to relax and let go.

How long?

There is no straight answer as to how long you stay in trance, but 15-20 minutes twice a day works just fine for most people. If you have a very busy schedule like most of us, perhaps you may prefer to do one longer session, say 30 – 40 minutes in the morning or evening. As you become more skilled at going into trance, you can practise it anywhere, on the train, in the park, at the office, on a plane, even standing up. You can go into trance for just a few minutes to relax yourself, or to change your mental state.

Sit or lie down.

When you first start using trance, it is best to find a quiet comfortable place where you will not be disturbed. You may sit or lie down, but

I recommend sitting down in a comfortable chair with your hands on your thighs and your feet flat on the floor. Lying down can produce very deep relaxation and does work well for some people, but, the problem is that you are more likely to fall asleep, especially if you are tired. Try experimenting with both ways, and find what works best for you.

Stress control - make or break.

If you are serious about controlling your weight, you have to be serious about controlling the stress in your life.

The great advantage to using self-hypnosis for losing weight (or for anything else) is the wonderful quality of relaxation that comes with trance.

Self-hypnosis has been used for years as a highly effective stress-management tool.

The natural simple act of entering a trance state has a profound healing effect on our mind and body. Brain wave activity changes, and harmful stress-producing chemicals are reduced. There is a release of tension in the body and all our beliefs (negative and positive) are temporarily suspended.

It is a very restful peaceful state in which our mind and body have time to heal and re-charge themselves.

I believe that man's number one goal should be to live life stress-free. The pure intention of trying to achieve this way of being will greatly improve the quality of one's life.

The great hypnotherapist Milton Erickson believed that we should live life with one foot in the present, and one foot in the future, I agree. Most of us go through life with one foot in the past and one foot in the future.

Regular trance sessions along with exercise, sensible eating, and a positive mental attitude will go a long to helping you stay stress-free, and will move you closer to your weight-loss goals.

Fake Motivation

Before you proceed with the exercises in this book, you need to ask yourself, do I really want to lose weight? This may sound strange to you initially, but think about it. Why do you want to lose weight?

All success in weight or fat-loss comes from your own motivated self. You have got to be 100% committed to your goal and you have to really want it. Some people try weight-loss programmes because they feel they should or because of social pressure. Perhaps they do it to please a loved one. This does not work. You must have true desire to reach your goal with 100% commitment.

*"I never worry about diets;
the only carrots that
interest me are the number
you get in a diamond"*

Mae West

2. High energy living.

Although this book is a book about losing weight through self hypnosis, it would be a crime to leave out some important basic facts regarding your bodies needs to function in a optimum way that is conducive to permantly controlling your weight. In the past I have tried many nutritional approaches and I have found it all boils down to a few simple facts that I would like to share with you now.

Carbs are king!

Carbohydrates are the foods that give us energy and should play a large part in your daily eating pattern. It is important though that you eat the right kinds.

Refined Carbohydrates

Refined carbs are the kind you need to keep to a minimum. Refined carbs contain high levels of white sugar and should be considered treats.

Examples are ....
White bread
Cakes
Chocolate
Jams
Biscuits

Fizzy drinks

Most breakfast cereals

Diets high in these foods will produce low energy levels, tiredness, and lack of motivation, and in the long term poor health!

Overall too many of these foods do not make for a healthy lifestyle and should be eliminated as much as possible.

Unrefined carbohydrates.

Including these carbs in your daily eating programme will make your weight loss goals even easier and will make you feel alive. These type of carbs also play a big part in the longevity and health of your mind and body.

Introducing more of these carbohydrates into your daily meals will help you to achieve your weight goals with an abundance of extra energy.

Examples…..

Brown rice

Pasta (whole wheat)

Potatoes

Wholemeal bread

Wholegrain cereals

Vegetables

Fresh fruit

Proteins – The building blocks of life.

An important ally to carbohydrates is protein. Protein plays a vital role in the function of all body cells and helps to build and maintain muscle tissue. Contrary to popular belief you do not need large amounts of it. You can get your daily needs by eating one medium portion of the following foods....

Fish
Chicken
Meat
Eggs
Cheese

Good fats.

We need fat for survival. It would be unhealthy and undesirable to have zero fat in our daily diet. It would also be very difficult as there is fat in many foods. It is important though to choose the right type of fat to help our bodies to function at an optimum level.
Try to avoid saturated and hydrogenated fats whenever possible. There is plenty of evidence to suggest that these are harmful to your health. Instead choose oils such as.....

Olive oil (extra virgin)

Flax oil

Sunflower oil

Using these oils in your diet will help you to live a more active, healthier and longer life.

The magic nutrient

As we are made up of over 75% water we need lots of it. Water is the number one nutrient, without it we can't survive. Water is the most important substance known to man.

Only oxygen is more vital to our survival. Forgetting to drink water is like forgetting to breath. Water is vital to your weight-loss success as it has no calories, cholesterol, or fat. Drinking water helps your kidneys function properly and in turn helps your liver to do one of its most important jobs of metabolising fat. So make sure you include 6-10 glasses a day as part of your eating programme.

"If you care enough for a result you will most certainly attain it"

-William James

3. Getting Started - Set your goals.

Have you ever packed your bags, got in your car, started the engine and driven onto the motorway and kept driving, not knowing where you were going, until you ran out of petrol? Of course not! That would be stupid! Yet that's exactly what millions of people do every day with regards to losing weight. Their goals are vague, with no real commitment behind them. So give yourself some time to sit down and decide what your ideal weight is, and when you would like to be at that weight.

Make sure the time frame is realistic. Don't try to lose more than 1-2 lbs of fat a week, because if you do, it will be more water than fat. You won't look good and you will feel lousy. As a rule 1-2lbs a week is plenty for lasting weight-loss.

Preparation.

Before you begin practising self-hypnosis follow these steps to ensure success.

Ask yourself, are you ready to make a 100% commitment to reaching your ideal weight? Are you doing it for yourself?
Write down the weight you desire to become. Is it realistic for you? Would it be your true ideal weight? Will you be able to comfortably maintain it?

Ask yourself, am I prepared to find 30 minutes to 40 minutes a day, five to six days a week to practice self-hypnosis?

Make sure you have the support of your family and friends. Tell them that you have made a commitment to reaching your goal. This will help you.

Moving more – Eating less.

All commercial diets have one major thing in common. They trick you into eating fewer calories and remind you to exercise more. The result is you lose weight. All these diets work through will power that at best produces a quick fix.

As we have discussed, 95% of diets fail at achieving long term results. Will power is not the answer for losing weight and keeping it off.

Inner changes

As you begin to relax, increase your awareness and learn to accept yourself unconditionally. You will find yourself making better lifestyle choices. You eat what you feel like eating, though after a short period of time you will find you choose to eat healthier, smaller amounts of food. Your desire for exercise increases. You will be more in tune with your body and its true needs. However before these changes come, you will need to consciously begin a sensible eating and exercise plan.

Follow these simple rules for maximum results:

1 Always eat what you feel like eating and keep junk food to a minimum. Aim to eat healthy nutritious food

2. Eat 25% less food than you normally would eat.

3. Try eating 5 smaller meals a day. This is much easier than it sounds. Eat breakfast, lunch, dinner, plus 2 x snacks such as fruit etc....

4. Increase your activity. Walk an extra 45 minutes a day on top of what you normally do. This can be broken down into 3 x 15 minute walks. Try walking instead of taking the car, bus or tube. Or you may prefer a long morning or evening walk.

Note. When you walk, walk briskly.

5. Drink lots of fresh clean, pure water. 6-10 glasses per day. This may be the magic nutriments for losing weight.

How to turbo charge your weight loss.

Buy a pedometer and work out how many steps you take each day for one week. Then gradually increase them. Try resistance training twice a week. This will increase your muscle tone and it is a great way of burning fat.

In just a short while you will find these simple changes integrating into your daily life, almost hypnotically as your regular trance sessions develop.

"Mind power is an actual living force"

- William Walker Atkinson

4. 42 Ways to Change.

(a) Trance Inductions
Breathe and relax.

The moment we were born we took a deep breath.

How often do we do that now?

To properly relax and be able to practise the exercises in this book you first need to learn deep diaphragmatic breathing. This is used in yoga and learning this alone will give you a powerful life tool to manage stress.

Exercise…

Put one hand slightly below your rib cage (just above the stomach)

Take a deep breath in through your nose and at the same time gently push out your stomach.

Hold for 3-4 seconds and then slowly breathe out through your mouth.

Repeat this three times and notice how you feel.

This can be practised any time anywhere as a way of developing instant calmness and is the correct way to breath before using self- hypnosis.

You will notice with some practice your breath will become fuller and longer.

Always make sure your stomach expands as you breathe in.

Mind and body relaxation technique.

Sit or lie down and make sure you will not be disturbed.

Close your eyes and take some deep breaths. Tune into the natural feeling of your breath. Don't try to change your breathing. Just gently become aware of the natural rise and fall of your chest............

Suggest to yourself that you are relaxing deeply. Focus your attention on the muscles on top of your head. Allow those muscles to soften, letting that comfort spread across your face, around the tiny muscles in your eyelids, into your neck and across your shoulders...............

Imagine comfort and ease spreading into your arms, hands and fingers................

Imagine that comfort spreading through the whole of your body from the top of your head all the way down to the tips of your toes...as you drift....deeper and deeper into relaxation with each soft natural breath you take.

Allow your mind to explore pleasant scenes in your imagination, using sounds, feelings, images..........in your own time slowly count up to 5 suggesting to yourself that you are becoming more and more aware and alert.

On 5 open your eyes and become fully aware.

Count yourself into trance technique.

Sit or lie down and allow your body to relax.

Take some deep breaths, breathing out any stress or tensions. Now slowly count up to 100 visualising each number as you count. When you reach 100 slowly count back, backwards.........

Imagine yourself relaxing more deeply with each number you count. As you reach 1 let yourself drift into a deep comfortable trance. Allow your mind to drift to pleasant scenes in your imagination.

In your own time drift back to full awareness, feeling relaxed and refreshed

Total relaxation.

Sit or lie down, take some deep breaths and give yourself permission to relax...................

Gently bring your awareness to your breathing and tune into the natural rhythm of your breath without trying to control it.

Just follow the natural rise and fall of your chest......

Begin to focus on the top of your head. Imagine all the muscles letting go allowing a pleasant wave of comfort to spread across your forehead, and around the tiny muscles of your eyelids, into your jaw all the way down into your neck and across your shoulders...

As you continue to relax imagine you have no bones in your arms, no bones in your hands and fingers. Just let your arms hang loosely down by your sides..................

Imagine you have no bones in your legs, your feet and toes. Just allow your legs to relax as you continue to relax more deeply into comfort..............

Gently bring your awareness to the top of your back. Imagine you have no spine, and allow your body to become limp loose and relaxed...

Find yourself relaxing more deeply with each soft easy breath you take.

Let your mind drift to pleasant scenes in your imagination, a relaxing beach, a peaceful meadow or perhaps a special peaceful private place that is right for you.............

Enjoy this special state of complete relaxation for a few minutes, and drift comfortably back to full awareness.

Visualisation.

Some people claim they can't visualise but the truth is everyone can visualise. Everything that exists in your life now, your car, your house, your partner, your career started as a mental image or movie.

When we desire something in our life we visualise it first (imagine it). We then attach emotion to it and then it becomes reality.

Try this exercise now.........

Close your eyes and imagine the front door of your house.

What colour is it?
As you open your front door what is the first thing you see?
What colour are the walls?
The floor?
You see my point.

Visualisation is simply using your imagination, and, when imagination is blended with desire and emotion, your goals will become reality.

Watch yourself in trance exercise.

Sit or lie down, close your eyes and take some deep breaths............

Imagine your body relaxing slowly from the top of your head all the way down to the tips of your toes...............

Now visualise, imagine yourself just as you are sitting or lying down. See yourself slowly relaxing into trance. Notice your breathing changing as you see yourself becoming more and more comfortable, your facial muscles relaxing, the comfortable position of your body, and, as you see yourself relaxing more deeply, you may notice the feelings of comfort and ease spreading through your body as you drift deeper and deeper into a relaxing trance.

The Betty Erickson technique.

This is one of my favourite hypnotic inductions.

Sit comfortably in a chair with your hands resting on your thighs, and allow yourself to relax for a few minutes.

Focus your eyes on a spot on the wall, or something of interest, a vase or maybe something reflective, a picture on the wall perhaps.

As you do this, say to yourself three statements about what you can see. e.g.…...

" I am aware of the reflection of the window in the vase"

" I am aware of the chair…….."

" I am aware of the picture frame ……"

Now 3 statements about what you can hear….e.g……..

" I am aware of the sound of the traffic…..the plane in the sky, the voices in the street….."

Now 3 statements about what you can feel e.g……..

" I am aware of my breathing, my hands resting on my thighs, my body becoming more and more comfortable…….."

Now 2 statements about what you can see, hear, and feel.

Now 1 statement about what you can see, hear and feel.

As you continue to relax allow your eyelids to close and tune into the feelings of comfort, spreading though your body, as you begin to direct the trance in whatever way you desire.

Arm Levitation.

Sit comfortably with your hands resting lightly on your thighs.

Make sure your fingertips are just making contact with the material of your clothes.

As you sit there look at your hands and wonder which hand will begin to lift up......

Will your right hand begin to float up or perhaps your left hand will begin to lift ...

Notice one of your hands beginning to feel lighter. As one of your hands lifts, find yourself relaxing more comfortably. Imagine a helium filled balloon is tied to your wrist. Imagine it pulling your arm upwards as your other hand and arm become heavier and heavier, and as the other arm becomes heavier suggest to yourself that when your lighter arm floats up and touches your face your eyelids close down and you drift into a deep comfortable trance....

As you continue to relax direct the trance as you desire.

Anchoring (The fist technique).

Once you have mastered the general trance techniques in this chapter, you can learn to go into hypnosis quickly and easily through the power of anchoring.

Relax into trance using one of the induction techniques. When you have achieved a deep comfortable state, focus your attention on one of your hands. Slowly bring that hand into a tight fist, becoming aware of the tension developing in your hand and forearm. As the tension increases mentally count to three in your mind. After the count of 3 slowly relax your hand....

Imagine a wave of comfort spreading up your arm, into your neck, shoulder and through the rest of your body.... Suggest to yourself that each time you do this (providing you are in a safe comfortable place) you will drift down into a pleasant, comfortable, relaxing trance.

Now slowly drift back to full awareness and test the anchor by forming a tight fist, mentally counting to three and then relaxing your hand. You will find that with a little practice you will be able to enjoy instant self-hypnosis.

"The mind directs the breath, letting it sink down, thereby penetrating even the bones"

-Yu –Seong Wu

(b) Awareness.

Self- awareness 1.

How often do we take the time to tune into what's going on inside our own bodies, our thoughts, feelings, sensations.

Self- awareness is an important key to understanding our feelings and emotions which play a big part in controlling our weight.

Try this exercise.

Sit down comfortably with your hands resting on your thighs.

Don't worry about going into trance, simply close your eyes and tune into your breathing, the natural rise and fall of your chest.

Don't try to alter your breathing just watch your breath. It may be shallow or perhaps very deep. It does not matter. Simply focus on the natural flow.

After a short while you will find your mind wandering, to what you were doing the previous day, what you must do later, what you must do next week.

This is normal so just gently bring your attention back to the breath.

As you continue to watch your breath, notice the beginning and the end of each breath.

The more you practice this natural meditation the more focused and aware you will become.

Practice for 10 – 15 minutes.

This can also be used as a trance induction.

Self- awareness 2.

Sit comfortably with your hands on your thighs.

Gently bring your attention to your breathing, as your mind begins to settle.

Tune into any sounds you are hearing around you, and gently bring your awareness to any body sensations, the weight of your arms, the sensations of your feet making contact with the floor.

Go into your body and tune in to any tensions, aches, and pains.

Don't make judgements - simply be aware.

Anytime you find your attention has wandered just gently bring it back to the breath.

Continue this exercise for 10-15 minutes.

Hypnotic Eating.

Here is a great exercise to help you start really tasting and enjoying your food. Eating awareness is crucial in learning to eat just the right amount of food your body needs. Remember digestion starts in your mouth. With just a little practice you will find yourself enjoying your food more, and eating only what your body needs.

As you sit down to eat take a deep breath, pick up your knife and fork and slowly bring the food to your mouth. As the food connects to your lips, become aware of the texture as it enters your mouth. Focus on the temperature of the food. Is it warm, cool, or hot? Wonder about the different colours as the food mixes in your mouth. While you eat, eat slowly, being mindful of every movement and sensation as you chew each mouthful. The experience is truly hypnotic.

"If you cannot find the truth right where you are, where else do you expect to find it"

\- Ralph Waldo Emerson

(c) Acceptance.

Self- Acceptance.

To be able to make lasting changes in ourselves we need to fully and completely accept ourselves unconditionally.

There is a certain magic about self-acceptance. It does not reinforce negative behaviour, but rather helps to permanently eliminate it.

Self-acceptance is part of the self-esteem concept and lies at the core of successful permanent weight- loss.

Exercise.......

Stand in front of a full length mirror (naked is best) and look at yourself. I don't mean your clothes. I mean you.

The shape of your body, your hair and face.

Acknowledge what you don't like about yourself and then accept it.

You may find it uncomfortable (to begin with) but stay with it.

When you find something you don't like (e.g. "my legs are too big, my face is too fat") just look into the mirror and say to yourself......

I accept myself fully, completely and unconditionally. Look into your eyes; look closely at the features of your face, your nose, mouth and ears.

Accept yourself fully and completely.

Do this exercise evening morning or night for 3-5 minutes.

Try it for 14 days; you may surprise yourself at the results.

Self–Focusing.

For thousands of years Eastern religions have known the power of the mantra.

A mantra is a sound, word or perhaps a series of words that is repeated silent or out loud to ones self.

This technique is an excellent way to focus and control the mind and can create powerful states of inner calm. The approach I want to teach you utilises your own name, and is an excellent way of developing self -acceptance and inner harmony.

Exercise

Find a comfortable chair sit down and relax. Take some deep breathes and focus your attention on your breathing. As you exhale silently repeat your name. This may seem strange at first, even slightly weird, but stay with the exercise, become completely absorbed in your name. If you find your mind drifting just gently bring yourself back to the sound of your name. Practice this meditation for 10-15 minutes a day over a three week period.

Energy Mirror.

Sit down.

Close your eyes and allow yourself to relax.

Imagine soft comfortable feelings spreading through your body.

Take a deep breath and breathe out any tensions.

Imagine looking at yourself in a full length mirror. As you notice parts of your body you don't like send love energy and approval to those parts.

Fill that energy with acceptance and reassurance for the way they are.

Imagine the energy as colours and shapes accept your body fully and completely.

"Our self image, strongly held essentially determines what we become"

- **Maxwell Maltz**

(d) Self Image.

Self image exercise.

How do you see yourself? What is your internal self-image like?

At the core of many weight problems lies a negative self-image. We all have our own internal blueprint of how we see ourselves.

This blueprint or self-image is formed through our own beliefs.

The person who stores a fat self-image will always claim to love junk food, have no time for exercise, or say they will start next week.

This mental blueprint may be out of our conscious awareness but it`s there, ready to be changed.

Here is a simple yet very effective exercise to help change your self-image.

Relax deeply into trance and create an image of yourself.

See yourself at your ideal weight looking happy, confident, slim, fit and healthy.

Notice how clear your skin is, see yourself wearing the clothes you love to wear.

Take your time …..

When you are happy with what you see, step into the image.

Imagine yourself being in the image, make sure it feels as good as it looks, tune into the positive feelings of living life at your ideal weight. Step out of the image. Make the image bigger and brighter, bring it closer and step into it again.

Connect to the feelings.

Repeat this exercise several times and drift up from trance with a sense of achievement, fully refreshed and fully aware.

Slim feelings self image.

Here is a powerful technique I use with my clients utilising kinaesthetics (feelings) to influence the subconscious mind.

Exercise…..

Accept yourself deeply in trance, and tune into how you feel at your present weight, the way your clothes feel against your skin, the heaviness of your arms and legs.

Notice any emotions that may present themselves………………

Continue to explore those body and mind feelings………………..

Now imagine you are 5lbs lighter. How does it feel being 5lbs lighter?

Tune into the feelings……………..

Continue the exercise by imagining you are 7lbs lighter and now imagine yourself at your ideal weight.

How do your clothes feel against your skin? Notice how you perhaps feel lighter psychologically as well as physically.

Continue with this excersie for 5-10 minutes and then slowly count up from one to five, suggesting to yourself at five you will be fully aware and wide awake.

Note…. This exercise may be broken down into smaller steps eg… 3lbs, 5lbs, 8lbs,10lbs until you reach your ideal weight.

*"I never resist temptation
because I have found
that things that are bad for me
do not tempt me"*

- George Bernard Shaw

(e) Weight Loss and Stress Control Strategies.

Get a worry Book.

One way to create stress is to constantly worry.

Worry creates anxiety and too much anxiety could well sabotage your weight-loss efforts.

One useful trick is to get a worry book. Carry a small notebook around with you. Every time you start to worry take out your note book and write your worry or concern down.

Think about whether you can take any immediate action to resolve this issue.

If you can, do it. If you can't, put your concern into the book and temporally suspend the worrying.

Later in the evening look at the book and give your self some time perhaps 10/15 minutes to meditate on how and when these concerns can be dealt with.

Change your Mind and Relax.

Whenever you find yourself feeling anxious or stressed, try the following exercise.

Sit comfortably and focus on your breathing.

As you begin to relax, notice where the negative images are in your mind.

They may be directly in front of you or perhaps to your right or to your left.

They may be movies or still pictures.
Notice whether they are in colour or black and white.

Do the pictures have sound?

If they have what is the tonality like?

Are you talking to yourself in a worried anxious way?

Are you shouting at yourself?

As the images get bigger, do you find yourself becoming more and more stressed?

Now here is the fun part.

Shrink the images and make them dimmer and send them out into the distance so they look like tiny dots.

As you do this turn down the volume (if there is any sound). Now replace these images with more calmer, peaceful pictures.

Soften your internal voice and slow it down.

Experiment with different tonalities.

Try voice tones that are the opposite of sounding stressed, anxious or angry.

Example... Talking to yourself in a calm peaceful almost seductive tone can be a powerful way of changing your internal state.

Experiment and find out what works for you.

Notice how by changing internal images and tonality you can dramatically change the way you feel.

No time for stress.

One way of looking at stress is that it is a fear, worry or concern relating to the past or the future.

This next exercise will help you feel better about a future event that you may feel anxious about.

Take your self into trance and imagine your future out in front of you.

Visualise or sense a time track.

Imagine floating forward in time to 20 minutes after the positive conclusion of the event you used to feel anxious about.

Stop and notice how your feelings have changed.

Look back and ask yourself. "Where has the anxiety all gone?"
Float back to the present and drift back to full awareness again. Now try to feel anxious about the time in which you thought you felt anxious.

How do you feel about the future event now?

Write to your unconscious.

Here is a great technique that will help you to create a new slimmer healthier self-image.

Sit down and write a short paragraph saying how you want to look and feel at your ideal weight.

Then condense it down into a single sentence, or just a word. Make sure you are happy with what you have written and that it is what you want.

Now roll the paper up into one of your hands, and go into trance.

Ask your unconscious for help in becoming this.

As you drift deeper into trance focus on the words in your hand, allow images, sounds and feelings to drift through your mind.....................

Drift up from the trance feeling wide awake and refreshed.

Emotional eating.

Are you an emotional eater? Do you eat when you are sad, bored, lonely, stressed or upset?

Let's take a look at how to identify between true physical hunger and emotional hunger. Physical hunger starts and builds up gradually beginning below the neck in the stomach approximately every three hours, and leads to a feeling of satisfaction after eating.

Emotional hunger begins suddenly above the neck with a craving for sweet or fatty foods. When given into it leads to feelings of guilt and shame.

Here is a powerful exercise to help you break the pattern of emotional eating forever.

Step 1. When you recognise the signals of emotional hunger, sit down and close your eyes and tune into the feelings.

Step 2. Recognise the inappropriate desire to eat.

Step 3. Feel the present emotion.

Step 4. What else can you feel?

Step 5. What specifically does this remind you of?

Step 6. Search for the pattern.

Positive motivation trigger.

Here is an exercise to really boost your motivation.

Close your eyes, take some deep breaths and relax. Allow yourself to drift into trance, and go back to a time when you felt totally motivated to do something that was important to you, and as you go back see what you saw, feel what you felt, and hear what you heard.

Watch yourself in the highly motivated state. Notice your posture, your voice tonality. Make the image big and bright and step into it.

Connect with the feelings. As you do this gently squeeze your thumb and index finger together. As the feelings begin to fade release your finger and thumb.

Now step out of the image, make it even bigger, brighter and step into it again.

Squeeze your thumb and index finger together as you experience the feelings

When the feelings begin to fade, release your thumb and finger and let your mind become clear.

Now just gently squeeze your thumb and finger together. You will feel the feelings of motivation spreading through your body.

If you do not feel the positive feelings you need to go back and repeat the exercise.

When you have successfully made the connection between the feelings and the thumb and finger squeeze, drift back up to full awareness again.

Anytime in the future you feel you need more motivation, just simply squeeze your thumb and finger together.

You can add more power to this exercise by adding a word or statement to the thumb/finger squeeze e.g...... As your thumb and finger connect say to yourself **"Do it now"** or **"Re-charge"**- anything that matches your experience.

For best results you should re-enforce this trigger by practising it each day.

This is a great technique for increasing your motivation to exercise. **DO IT NOW!**

Weight loss strategy.

Here is a technique based on the work of the great hypnotherapist Milton Erickson.

Milton used to tell his weight loss clients to buy only enough food for one day. They must walk to the food store and back each day. This achieved two things.

The walking provided excellent fat burning exercise, and the daily shop developed a sense of control over eating.

If you are willing to commit to this excellent strategy you can really turbo charge your results. I have personally used this approach with my own clients and believe me it really works.

To help you create this new behaviour, go deeply into trance and visualise yourself doing this over and over until it seems like it is happening now.

Decision Delay Technique.

Can you think of a time when you had a desire to eat or drink something, then after a short period of time you just lost all interest?

Most of us have had this experience at some time in our life. This is usually because we have given ourselves enough time for our awareness to let us know that perhaps we don't really need what it was that we desired.

Here is a psychological technique that could help you avoid eating literally hundreds of empty calories a day.

When you find yourself craving something sweet or fatty, a desert, or a perhaps a craving for a late night snack, look at your watch and note the time. Tell yourself that you will suspend your decision to indulge in the food or drink for a period of 20 minutes and commit to it. Then after 20 minutes go in side and ask yourself, do I really want this glass of wine, or piece of chocolate? (Or whatever).

You may be surprised how your feelings have changed.

Try Something Different.

When I begin hypnotherapy with a new client, I often will tell them to make one small change in their life.

This could be something as simple as joining a health club. The point is, small changes can and do lead to bigger changes, so as soon as you begin to work towards your new weight-loss goal try doing something different in your life.

Here are some ideas….
Drive a different way to work
Walk a different way to work
Join a new club or group
Take up gardening
If you don't like your job, find a new one.
Join a new health club

Get creative and make a change.

Past Resources.

Probably the easiest way to utilise trance is to simply ask you're unconscious what you want it to do then go into trance and let it happen.

Exercise...

Sit down comfortably and take some deep breathes.

Allow yourself to relax for a few minutes.

Say to yourself….

"I would like my unconscious to go back into my past and replay with sounds, feelings and images the three times when I have been highly motivated and focused on eating sensibly and being more physically active."

Then have those behaviours occur spontaneously and naturally at the appropriate times in the future …

Now take yourself into trance using any method you choose and just allow thoughts, feelings, and images to drift through your mind without any conscious effort.

After 15/20 minutes drift back to full awareness with a sense of achievement.

Reframing.

There is always more than one way to look at things.

Some people seem to enjoy finding the negatives of a situation, whilst others tend to look at the positive side.

When somebody describes a situation in a negative sense, and somebody then points out the positive side, this is called reframing.

You can utilise this wonderful technique to help you reach your weight loss goals.

e.g..."I hate exercise" .....Re-frame...." I hate being fat even more. Exercise can help me become slimmer and happier."

e.g..."I have spent half my life trying different diets without success"..... Re-frame... "But it has helped me find out what really works"......Simple isn't it.

The next time you find yourself thinking negatively about your weight loss goals, reframe it.

The more you do this the more you will automatically tend to choose a more positive point of view.

Reframing is also a very useful tool for controlling stress, by looking at negative situations from a different perspective.

You can change the way you feel about almost anything.

Mental rehearsal.

To achieve a new goal we have to be first able to do it inside our minds. If you run a mental movie of your goal often enough it will become your reality.

Psychologists have been teaching these techniques for many years. Athletes have been practising them for centuries

Make mental rehearsal part of your daily self-hypnosis and watch yourself change.

Exercise…

Relax yourself comfortably into hypnosis using any technique you choose.

Take your time to develop your trance.

Imagine yourself doing the things you need to do to reach your goal ie…..

Exercising, walking, eating less, choosing healthier foods etc….

Run a movie using sounds, feelings and full colour.

It is important you use your three main senses or even all five of them, sounds, feelings, pictures, taste, and smell.

This will make the imagery more real, and more powerful.

Run the movie again and again until you feel confused as to whether you are imagining the future or experiencing the past.

Slowly return back to full awareness again.

Visual food elimination.

Mental images are powerful we are constantly making pictures to match our thoughts and words.

To know what you want in life you have to visualise it.

Although much of this is unconscious we can control these images at the conscious level if we so desire.

Here is a good exercise for taking control of your own internal images to help you to choose the right kind of foods that will help you achieve your ideal weight.

Exercise....

Close your eyes and relax yourself completely into trance any way you choose.

Bring up an image of some chocolate, cake, crisps or other food you find hard to resist.

Make the image clear, big and bright in your mind.

Imagine it in front of you.

Now put a large black X in the middle of the picture, make the X big and clear.

When you have the black X covering the whole of the image, shrink the image down to a size of a postage stamp.Drain the colour and send it into the distance so it looks like a tiny dot. (Do this fast)

Repeat this 5-10 times and then try to get the image back. How has it changed?

How do you feel about that food now?

If you find you can still easily hold onto the image repeat the exercise until you no longer connect to the picture.

You can repeat this with any food you want to stop eating.

After you have done this start to visualise your favourite healthy foods big, bright and colourful in front of you

See yourself enjoying these new healthier foods.

Come back to full awareness, relaxed and refreshed.

Chocolate addiction buster.

For all you people who say you can't stop eating chocolate, here is a very powerful technique for stopping it now!

Sit or lie down. Don't worry about going into trance as it will happen naturally as you do the exercise. Close your eyes and make an image of your hands full of chocolate (seeing it from your own eyes). Make the image clear and bright in your mind and make sure you focus on the chocolate.

The background of the image should be of somewhere where you normally eat chocolate e.g. Kitchen, dining room etc…

Alright. Now move that image to your left. We will come back to it later.

Now create another image (looking at yourself). See yourself looking healthy fit happy and confident at your ideal weight,

Make sure you really like what you see – this is important.

Make it big and bright and colourful. Take some time on this. When you are completely happy with what you see bring the first image (the chocolate image) back.

Put this in front of you with the positive self image behind it.

You should now just see the chocolate, image in front of you. The positive image should be behind it.

As you focus on the chocolate make a hole in the middle of the image.

As you do this allow the positive self image to pour through completely covering the chocolate image.

Do this really fast five times, and let your mind clear.

Now try to get the first image back (the chocolate one). Already this may seem difficult.

Repeat the exercise again, this time doing it ten times even faster and let your mind clear. Try to get the first image back and find it difficult.

Repeat this exercise until you can only see the positive you at your ideal weight.

Practice this everyday until you lose the desire to eat chocolate.

Important – Make sure you are in the first image (associated) and looking at yourself in the second image (disassociated)

Self Talk.

"I will never be slim"

"I hate exercise"

"I will try to stop eating chocolate"

"All the women in our family are overweight"

If you were to practice just one psychological technique for losing weight, I would strongly suggest changing your internal dialogue.

As you read the first paragraph you may have found some of those statements familiar.

People who go through life struggling with their weight often practice the wrong kind of self-talk.

Negative self-talk will almost always sabotage any weight loss programme.

Negative internal dialogue will only help reinforce a negative self-image.

Consider the following statements.

"The more I exercise the more slimmer I become. As each day passes I find my desire for eating healthy natural foods increases. I enjoy eating just the right amount of food that my body needs"

Get into the habit of speaking to yourself in a way that will help move you towards your chosen goal. Use present tense language "I am becoming slimmer, I enjoy eating just the right amount of food my body needs. Exercise makes me feel great" Get the idea?

Remember...... Self-talk is a natural form of self-hypnosis. Programme yourself for success.

Change your T words.

When I listen to people talk about their weight loss challenges, I hear many people making negative statements. They say things like...

"I can't motivate myself to walk more"

"I can't stop eating"

Whether you think you can or can't, you are right because they're your beliefs, your words.

If you are guilty of this way of thinking try the following exercises...

Write down all the things you say that you can't do.

e.g........

"I can't eat less food"

"I can't drink more water"

Now opposite these statements write down....

"I won't eat less"

"I won't drink less water"

How do you feel about these statements now?

The truth is you chose not to do these things.

Once you can accept this reality you can start to lose the "t" off of the word "can't" and then you can!

Indirect Suggestions for Weight Loss.

Go into a deep comfortable trance and wonder to yourself....

"When will I begin to eat less chocolate?" (Or whatever you overindulge in)

"Perhaps I will remember to eat just at meal times and remember to forget at other times."

And I wonder how my unconscious will help me find other new creative ways of eating less and moving more"

These suggestions are indirect and allow your unconscious/ subconscious mind to search for ideas and solutions, utilising your own inner resources.

Pattern break.

One of the biggest challenges of losing weight is changing patterns of behaviour.

The easiest way to change an unwanted pattern is to do something completely different.

This can be done by shocking our nervous system, by acting in a different way. By using our sensory system in a new way we can create amazing changes.

Instead of looking for the "why" of a problem, the key is looking to create new patterns of behaviour through being creative and flexible.

Experiment with the following exercises....

Every time you feel a strong urge to snack on the wrong foods, make it a rule that you always use your non-dominant hand (if right handed use your left). This is a very simple way of breaking up an unwanted pattern of behaviour.

You can take this a step further. Every time you feel a strong urge to binge or snack on junk food, make it a rule that you put on your best shirt or top first. Then with your non-dominant hand continue the binge or snack. You will be amazed at how different you feel about the food.

Interrupt your Pattern.

Can you think of a time when you were expecting to binge on chocolate or junk food, then for some reason you didn't.

Perhaps you got distracted by a phone call or you become engrossed in an interesting book or maybe you decided to go to the gym.

The key here is not to try to understand why you did not do it but what you did to interrupt the pattern.

Focus on the alternative behaviour and use it as a solution.

If your binges or times of overeating are usually in the evening, and in the past have been avoided by going to see a friend or going out for a walk, start to think about how you can introduce these positive interruptions into your life on a regular basis as a powerful weight control strategy.

Make your future real.

Here is a secret that will help you lose weight and keep it off.

Slim people project themselves into the future and imagine all the negatives of over-eating. They tune into the feelings of what it would be like to be over- weight. This gives them an awareness of the consequences of overindulging. As a result they make better choices with regards to what they eat. This can also work well as a motivation for exercise. This can work for you too.

Exercise…

Go into trance any way you choose.

As you find yourself relaxing deeply imagine two crystal balls, one to your left and one to your right.

In one of the crystal balls visualise yourself five years into the future.

See an image of you who has not changed anything about your lifestyle. How much more do you weigh? What is the state of your health? Where is your level of happiness? What size clothes do you wear? How has your weight affected your life?

Take all the learning.

Now take a look at the other crystal ball.

See the "you" in five years time having been practicing self-hypnosis, exercising, eating sensibly.

How have you changed?

How is your weight, your clothes size, your health, your happiness? How do you feel - take all the learning.

Come back to this exercise every few weeks and focus more and more on your positive future and make it real.

Parts resolve.

Everybody has found themselves in conflict at some time in their lives.

"A part of me wants to go to the movies, but part of me wants to have a night in at home"

"Part of me wants to go on a diet, but part of me likes eating fatty foods"

As human beings we have many different parts to ourselves, sometimes referred to as ego states. Of course these parts or ego states don't exist on a physical level. They are our own personal inner states.

We have happy parts, sad parts, loving parts, motivated parts, lazy parts.

The list goes on.

Many clients that arrive at my practice have inner conflicts. This is especially true with weight problems.

What is normally required is a parts integration to resolve the conflict.

Exercise.....

Relax deeply into trance with your hands resting comfortably on your thighs, palms facing upwards.

Imagine putting the glutton part (or whatever) of yourself into one of your hands, and the opposite part, the part of you that wants to change into the other hand.

Tune into your hands and notice the differences in the two parts. Perhaps one is heavier or lighter than the other, maybe one part is a different shape or colour.

Now ask your unconscious to start a negotiation between the two parts. As you go deeper into trance, trust your unconscious to do its work.

As you focus on your hands allow them to slowly come together almost by themselves.

1. **2.**

3.

Parts Resolve

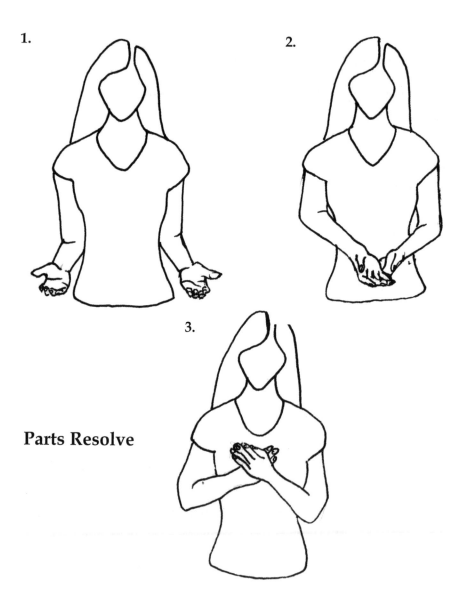

When both hands (parts) have come completely together, bring the parts back into your self as one integrated whole by bringing both hands to your chest.

Keep your hands on chest until you feel the integration is complete.

Slowly return back to full awareness with a glowing sense of achievement.

Note...... Allow yourself plenty of time for the parts to fully integrate.

A weight off your mind through metaphor.

One sure way of communicating with our unconscious is through the power of metaphor. We use metaphor all the time.

"He's a pain in the neck"

"I feel free as a bird"

"I am on top of the world"

Metaphor may well be the language of the unconscious. In modern hypnotherapy the use of story telling and symbolising is apparent. This is because analogies and metaphors work well at bypassing the conscious mind and are potent ways of creating change. You too can use this powerful hypnotic approach in your self-hypnosis.

Exercise.

Relax deeply into trance and tune into the feelings you hold with regard to reducing your weight.

Ask your unconscious to help you create a metaphor that represents your weight loss challenge.

Give it a form, it may be a shape, colour, object, building, tunnel, animal anything that fits for you.
As you explore your imagery find creative ways of changing the imagery into a more positive form.

A client of mine once told me she saw her weight problem as being locked up in a large iron safe. I told her to first wonder about the words – safe, heavy and combination. Do they symbolise anything of importance or not? Or is being "heavy" linked to feeling safe. Is a different combination of food required? Could she imagine opening the safe and learning even more about her weight concern, or even completely resolve it.

Whatever form your weight challenge takes, simply change it to a more positive metaphor that gives you more freedom and choice.

Put on a slim head.

Relax into trance and imagine yourself standing behind someone you know who has lost weight and has kept it off.

Make the image bright and colourful in your mind.

Now imagine reaching out and taking off their head and putting it on yours.

Take on that person's way of thinking with regards to losing weight and keeping it off.

Learn about their attitudes towards food and exercise.

As you wear their head learn about their beliefs and behaviours.

This is a truly powerful technique for creating change.

A Different Perspective.

Imagine being able to step outside of yourself and taking a look at yourself from a different perspective.

Being able to hear yourself talking about your weight control issues, watching yourself talking to friends about the way you feel about yourself.

I wonder how much you could learn about yourself.

Sit down and allow your body to relax letting go of any tensions as you become more and more comfortable.

Imagine watching yourself talking to friends or family about your weight concerns.

Hear your voice and notice the words and statements you make about your self.

See and hear yourself from a new perspective.
Notice the many different ways you have of responding to others.

Monkey see monkey do.

In the last decade neuroscientists have provided some incredible insights to how we learn and empathise with others.

Whenever we watch someone carry out a task or action of interest, mirror neurons are fired off in our brain, creating a rapid replay in our mind. These new insights are providing psychologists with interesting theories about human learning and behaviour.

So how can our mirror neurons help us lose weight and keep it off?

By modelling slim people we can learn to eat in the same way, exercise in the same or similar way, and also learn to think the same.

A good way to do this is to find someone you know who has lost weight and succeeded in keeping it off. Ask them how they achieved it. Ask them about their beliefs and attitudes towards food and exercise, about their behaviours and habits, how they stay slim.

Learn about their inner resources and then beg, steal or borrow them.

In a nutshell model them.

5. Food for thought.

Congratulations for finishing this book.

If you take the time to practice and develop the skills within these pages, you will own the power to control your weight and keep it off for life. You may even decide to attend one of my seminars to help you reach your ideal weight more quickly giving you the added advantage of receiving personal mind coaching. Whatever you decide please let me know about your successes.

Now here are the ten keys to losing weight and keeping it off.

1) Write down your goals
2) Self awareness
3) Acceptance
4) Change your self-image
5) Chew your food slowly
6) Eat 25% less food
7) Walk an extra 45 minutes per day (walking briskly)
8) Eat little and often 4-5 smaller meals – eat what you feel like eating
9) Drink plenty of water
10) Watch and learn the habits and behaviours of slim people

There you have it now it's up to you.
As the shoe people say **"Just do it"**

Further reading

Psycho–Cybernetics
– *Maxwell Maltz*

The six pillars of self esteem
– *Nathaniel Branden*

The step diet
Hill Peters Joutberg

To contact Marcus D'Silva go to

www.marcus-dsilva.com

email: info@marcus-dsilva.com